Guaranteed Weight Loss:

20 Healthy And Easy Crock Pot Recipes

Table of content

Introduction

Let's face it. You have a busy schedule. Losing weight and keeping it off is a challenge. Some recipes take too long when you just walk in the door from a hectic day. What is the solution?

This book consists of 20 recipes that are delicious, high in fat low in carbs can be made in the slow cooker. Now isn't that convenient? You assemble the ingredients and put them in the crock pot before you head to work or later if you have time. Dinner is ready without the stress. Get your taste buds ready. Don't give up you are on your way to becoming a good cook.

Chapter 1 – Soups and Chowder

This classic comfort food won't go to waste. You cannot go wrong with this soup unless there is a picky eater in the household like mine. I go for the standard. I have seen different ways to make this dish but I need easy and warm

Chicken noodle soup

Serves 8

Ingredients

8cups of water

4 medium sliced carrots

1 small chopped onion

2 bay leaves

1/2teaspoon dried thyme

 salt

 ground pepper

3 ½ lb whole chicken

3 cups of egg noodles (you can also use rotini pasta)

Directions

1. In a slow cooker that is 4 ½-6 quarts blend water, carrots, celery,onion, bay leaves, thyme, 4 tsp salt, and ½ tsp pepper. Put the chicken on the vegetables. Cover with the lid and cook as directed in the manual on low heat for 8-10 hours or high for 4-5 hours.

2. Place chicken on cutting board. Throw away bay leaves. Add the noodles to the crock pot; cover and cook an additional 20 minutes

3. As the noodles cook, peel, remove, and discard skin, fat, and leaves from chicken; shred meat with a fork

4. Skim fat with a spoon and throw away. Return chicken to pot and serve

This warming soup goes well with whole grain rolls or sourdough rolls. A sprinkling of thyme or parsley will add color to it. It takes less than four hours so perhaps you can start to prepare it in the afternoon in time for dinner.

Serves 6-8

This is another dish with a few variations. Feel free to use potatoes or bacon and chives if you want. I know one thing, that it is guaranteed nourishment and definitely a winner. You can have some crusty bread on the side too. I hope you will agree

Shrimp corn chowder

Ingredients

2 lbs shelled and deveined small shrimp

½ cup chopped onion

2 tsp butter

2 cans (12oz) evaporated milk

2 potatoes chopped

2 cups chicken broth

1 can white or sweet yellow corn (or frozen)

1tsp Creole seasoning

½ tsp garlic powder

2 T of all-purpose flour

Directions

1. Saute onion in butter until tender. In a 5 quart slow cooker combine onion, milk, creole seasoning, and garlic powder. Add everything else except for shrimp.

2. Put on the lid and cook on low for 3 hours. Next add the shrimp.

3. Stir. Cook an additional 30 minutes or until shrimp are heated through. If chowder is too thick add 1 cup of chicken broth

Note: If you do not have creole seasoning you can use the following spices1/4 tsp salt, garlic powder, and paprika, and a pinch of dried thyme, cumin, and cayenne pepper.

Low carb lunch or Sunday dinner, this will be a joy to prepare. Throw together these ingredients. Well, cutting the onions is hardest part. May I suggest goggles or lighting a candle so your eyes won't burn. Once that is over transfer them to the crock pot.

French Onion Soup

Serves 4

French bread

3 Tablespoons all-purpose flour

4 large thinly onions (red, yellow, or white)

3 gloves of garlic

6 cups fat free beef broth

8 thin slices of Gruyere or Swiss cheese

2 cups thinly sliced mushrooms

2 Tablespoons butter

2 teaspoons olive oil

Directions

1. Melt butter and heat oil in large frying pan at very low heat until they caramelize. This takes about 20 minutes

2. Add onions, garlic, Worcestershire, mushrooms to crock pot. Stir in flour and let cook for 5 minutes. Add broth and cook on low heat for 6-8 hours.

3. Now the good part: French bread on the soup and cover with Swiss or Gruyere- Broil for 3 minutes. Get bowls and spoons

Even though it's minus the meat, this vegetarian stew is sure to please. I am aware some folks do not like squash and the summer type may be out of season. With that in mind substitution is possible. Spinach or kale goes well with tortellini

Tortellini Tuscan Stew

Serves 6

Ingredients

1 butternut squash cut into chunks

1 lg zucchini cut, peeled, and seeded (chunks)

1 large yellow summer squash

1 large diced onion

1 large diced red pepper

4 oz thin green beans trimmed

1 can (28 oz) crushed tomatoes

2Tablespoon fresh chopped oregano

1 can chicken or vegetable broth

1 ½ teaspoon chopped garlic

¾ tsp salt

1 pkg cheese tortellini

1 bag(5oz) baby spinach

3Tablespoon grated Parmesan cheese

Directions

1. Put in all ingredients except tortellini. Cover and cook on high heat for 3 hours or on low 6 hours.

2. Remove the lid turn heat to high and stir in tortellini. Cover and boil 15 minutes until pasta is almost tender

3. Cover; cook 5 minutes until spinach has wilted and pasta is tender.

One of my favorite dishes. I could eat it everyday but that's just me. Bless the creator of this meal. This terrific comfort food is really creamy and spicy. If you have small children leave out the chipotle chile sauce. You can refrigerate the leftovers (That's if there are any)

Turkey Chili

Serves 6

1 T olive oil

1 large onion

20 oz ground turkey

2 C beef broth

1 15 oz can diced tomatoes

2 15 oz can black beans

1 15 oz refried beans

1 C salsa

2 T chili powder

1 T ground cumin

½ tsp cayenne

1T chipotle chile in adobo sauce

1 T tomato paste

salt and pepper

Shredded Mexican Blend or sharp cheddar cheese

Directions

1. Heat olive oil in a large pan

2. Toss in onion and saute for about 5 minutes until they soften

3. Add the onion and ground turkey to the crock pot

4. Put in the remaining ingredients and give it a stir

5. Cover with lid and allow it to simmer for 6 hours

6. Season to taste with salt and pepper

7. Garnish with cilantro and lime if you wish

Your taste buds and family (or guests will thank you).

In the past I have made the fried kind of this cuisine and I am fortunate to find a recipe with less grease and the right kind of fat. It comes kid approved . A restaurant quality meal. My mouth is watering from the memories. I can't use chopsticks yet but I am working on it.

Sweet n-Sour Chicken

Serves 4

¼ c rice vinegar

1 Tablespoon soy sauce

1 Table cornstarch

1 Tablespoon canola oil

3 Tab Orange Marmalade or 1 /4 cup pineapple juice, ¼ cup apple juice

2 Tablespoon ketchup

2 Tablespoon brown sugar

8 oz chicken breasts or tenders cut into bit-size pieces

1 garlic clove

2 teaspoon ginger (grated or minced)

½ cup of organic low sodium chicken breasts or homemade

1 cup broccoli florets

16 oz bag stir fry veggies

Pam Spray or olive oil

Optional:

brown rice or quinoa

Directions

1.Cook brown rice or quinoa according to package directions

2.Whisk orange marmalade or pineapple/apple juice, corn starch, vinegar, soy sauce, ketchup and brown sugar together.

3. Put stir fry veggies and broccoli, in crock pot; add the chicken.

4. Pour the reserved sauce over the meat

5. Put on the lid. Stir cornstarch into reserved liquid. Add to the pot

6. Cook and simmer on low heat for 4-5 hours. Turning the heat on high for the last 30 minutes.

7. Cook covered for additional 30 minutes until sauce is thickened. Serve on brown rice or quinoa

Chapter 2 – Sandwiches

Another seal of approval from the children. I made this meal out of desperation when I couldn't figure what to make with so few ingredients. I am glad I did and there was seconds. This is our permanent menu option for dinner.

Serves 6

Buffalo chicken wraps

24 oz skinless chicken breasts

1 stalk of celery

1/2 diced onion

1 garlic

16 oz fat free low sodium chicken broth

1/2 hot sauce (frank's)

For the wraps

Shredded lettuce

Shredded cheddar cheese

2Tablespoon ranch dressing

Directions

1. In crock pot add chicken, onions, celery stalk, garlic and enough broth to cover chicken. Put on lid and cook on high level for 4 hours

2. Take out the chicken use 1/2 cup of the broth and dispose of the rest. You can shred the chicken using two forks and put back in the slow cooker with the broth and hot sauce and set to high for 30 more minutes.

To make your wraps, lay down tortillas. Add chicken, then cheese, and finally ranch dressing. Roll up and eat.

Preparing this other white meat is simple when you use a slow cooker. Onion and pork merge with a savory sauce. Put the heat on low and the cooker finishes the job. The shredded meat is put on soft buns for a southern style fare.

Serves 16

Pulled Pork

Ingredients

1 medium onion chopped

½ cup apple cider vinegar

¼ cup light molasses

½ cup ketchup

2 Tablespoons sweet paprika

2 Tablespoons spicy brown mustard

2 Tablespoons Worcestershire sauce

1 teaspoon cayenne pepper

1teaspoon ground pepper

1 teaspoon salt

½ teaspoon hickory smoke flavoring (optional)

roast (pork butt) cut into 4 pieces

16 warm soft sandwich buns

Directions

1. Stir onion, vinegar, ketchup, molasses, paprika, mustard, Worcestershire, cayenne pepper, black pepper, salt and ¼ cup of water until blended. Add to the pork to the mixture and toss

2. Put the lid on and cook ingredients as directed in the instruction manual; about 8-10 hours

3. Take out pork and put into a bowl or cutting board. Pour sauce into a glass measuring cup or medium bowl. Proceed to shred pork with two forks . Put the shredded pork back into the slow cooker. Remove fat from the sauce and dispose of it. Pour sauce over pork and give it a good toss

4. Serve pork on buns. Enjoy

This classic always fills the belly with love and satisfaction. Instant happiness and one of the best dinners ever. It comes prepared with all the trimmings. Sit back and watch your family gobble up the juicy meat. Melt in your mouth goodness. Need I say more?

Pot roast

Serves 8

1 Tablespoon cornstarch

10 baby carrots

1 (3lb) beef chuck roast

2 T Worcestershire sauce

2 T A1 or any steak sauce

2 small Russet potatoes

1 onion

2 tsp Italian dressing

1 cup beef broth

salt and black pepper to taste

Directions

1.Mix 2 T of cold water and cornstarch. Whisk until smooth

2. Season roast with steak sauce, Worcestershire sauce, and Italian dressing and place in slow cooker.

3. Place carrots, onions, and around roast. Pour on beef broth. Simmer on low heat for 8 hours.

4. Let it rest fifteen minutes and then slice.

I know this is the sandwich section so you can make hot roast beef sandwiches on Kaiser rolls for leftovers.

Chapter 3 – Entrees

Even though it's minus the meat, this vegetarian stew is sure to please.

Tortellini Tuscan Stew

Serves 6

Ingredients

1 butternut squash cut into chunks

1 lg zucchini cut, peeled, and seeded (chunks)

1 large yellow summer squash

1 large diced onion

1 large diced red pepper

4 oz thin green beans trimmed

1 can (28 oz) crushed tomatoes

2Tablespoon fresh chopped oregano

1 can chicken or vegetable broth

1 ½ teaspoon chopped garlic

¾ tsp salt

1 pkg cheese tortellini

1 bag(5oz) baby spinach

3Tablespoon grated Parmesan cheese

Directions

4. Put in all ingredients except tortellini. Cover and cook on high heat for 3 hours or on low 6 hours.

5. Remove the lid turn heat to high and stir in tortellini. Cover and boil 15 minutes until pasta is almost tender

6. Cover; cook 5 minutes until spinach has wilted and pasta is tender.

This terrific comfort food is really creamy and spicy. If you have small children leave out the chipotle chile sauce. You can refrigerate the leftovers (That's if there are any)

Turkey Chili

Serves 6

1 T olive oil

1 large onion

20 oz ground turkey

2 C beef broth

1 15 oz can diced tomatoes

2 15 oz can black beans

1 15 oz refried beans

1 C salsa

2 T chili powder

1 T ground cumin

½ tsp cayenne

1T chipotle chile in adobo sauce

1 T tomato paste

salt and pepper

Shredded Mexican Blend or sharp cheddar cheese

Directions

8. Heat olive oil in a large pan

9. Toss in onion and saute for about 5 minutes until they soften

10. Add the onion and ground turkey to the crock pot

11. Put in the remaining ingredients and give it a stir

12. Cover with lid and allow it to simmer for 6 hours

13. Season to taste with salt and pepper

14. Garnish with cilantro and lime if you wish

Your taste buds and family (or guests will thank you)

Cedar Plank Salmon

Yes, you have to find a cedar plank to adjust and fit into your crock pot but it's worth it. Now you can give it a toasty smell and brown tone. To achieve this, burn it over an open flame on your stove. This is only a recommendation. Weigh it down with cans to soak for an hour or overnight. You go not have to dry it before use.

Serves 4

Ingredients

1 cedar plank

½ teaspoon salt

1 ½ lb salmon filet

1 sliced lemon

1 Tablespoon grainy mustard

2 T maple syrup or McCormick Grill mates Smokehouse Maple

1 T butter

1 tsp parsley (minced)

Directions

1. Put cedar plank into crock pot. Season salmon w/salt and pepper and McCormick Grill Mates and place on plank.

2. Put lemons on fish. Cook for 2 hours on low heat

3. Throw away lemon. Some white protein around the salmon is common

Skip the next step if using McCormick Grill Mates

4. Melt butter, mustard, and maple syrup   in the microwave. Pour onto salmon

5. Sprinkle some parsley and it's ready

Chapter 4 – Breakfasts

Included here are healthy breakfast for any day of the week. The most important meal of the day   includes fruits, veggies, bacon, or cheese. Whatever you crave. Protein is not a wild diet trend. You should not neglect it for your dietary needs. You can achieve a balance with moderation. It builds lean muscle. We lose it in our middle-age. Protein achieves that full feeling. If you eat if for breakfast you will eat less throughout the day.

20-30 grams are recommended.

Prepare this the night before and spend your free time waiting however you like. Relax. Do some laundry. Watch a movie while it simmers. It is chock full of bacon, eggs, cheese, and hash brown crispness.

Breakfast Casserole

Serves 8

1 lb bacon or turkey bacon

1 medium sweet onion

1 large red bell pepper

2 cup sharp cheddar cheese

1 dozen eggs

salt and pepper

1 package hashed browns

1 diced green onions

2 cups shredded Monterey jack

½ cup feta cheese

1 cup nonfat milk

1 teaspoon salt

1 ½ teaspoon pepper

Directions

1. These ingredients will be piled into 2 or 3 layers. Layer the hash browns. Next the turkey bacon, green onions, cheeses, peppers and onions

2. Whisk eggs , milk, salt, and pepper together

3. Pour into crock pot

4. Cover and cook on low heat 10 hours until eggs set and are no longer runny

I am an oatmeal lover. I learned how to make my own instead of relying on those processed packets. This is a vegetarian recipe. I don't wish to exclude anyone so use any alternate as you see fit. It's just yum . One of my all -time favorites.

Serves 4

Overnight Cinnamon Apple Oatmeal

Pam or another non-stick cooking spray

2 large chopped apples (Granny Smith or Pink Lady)

11/2 cup skim milk

1 1/2 cup water

1cup whole grain oats

3 Tab packed brown sugar

2 Tablespoon butter

1 Tablespoon cinnamon

2 Tablespoon ground flax seed

1/4 teaspoon kosher salt

Optional toppings

1/4 cup dried raisins or cranberries

1/4 cup chopped walnuts, almonds, pecans

Directions

1. Spray a 3 1/2 or bigger slow cooker with Pam cooking or other non-stick cooking spray.

2. Stir together chopped apples, milk, water, oats, sugar, butter, and flax. Cover with lid and cook on low heat for 7-8 hours or overnight. Add kosher salt to oatmeal before serving.

I recently discovered you can replace quinoa for oats. Great, right because I have a bunch of it. A warm bowl of deliciousness to begin your day. An instant nutritious breakfast. Experiment with this one too if it makes it easier on you. This yummy breakfast smells delicious. It digests easily

6 servings

Banana Bread Quinoa

1 cup quinoa

1/2 cup light cream

1/2 C low-fat milk

1 cup water

1 1/2 banana

2 Tablespoons chopped walnuts

3 Tablespoons brown sugar

1 1/2 Tablespoon melted butter

1/2 teaspoon vanilla extract

Directions

1. Use a fork to mash the banana in a bowl and put it aside. In another bowl blend walnuts and brown sugar

2. Pour quinoa, light cream, cinnamon, milk, water, butter and vanilla into the crock pot. Then add the banana to the mix and stir. Sprinkle the walnut and sugar into it and stir.

3. Simmer on low heat for 4-6 hours or until quinoa is done. You may add more liquid or sugar for flavor

Serve and top with sliced bananas for garnish

The smell of veggie goodness as you wake is one of life's pleasures. Tofu can go into these too. It is not a must. You will still be delighted by the taste and color. You can also skip the tortillas. Try it with avocado and sour cream.

Serves 6

Vegetarian Breakfast Burritos

Ingredients

1 15oz can of drained and rinsed black beans

1 10oz can diced tomatoes w/ green chiles

1 cup cooked barley

2 cup vegetable broth

3/4 cup frozen corn

1/4 cup chopped green onions

1 teaspoon ground cumin

1 teaspoon chili powder

1/2 teaspoon ground red pepper

3 chopped garlic cloves

Directions

1.Stir all ingredients into the crock pot and cook on low heat for 5 hours

2.After the filling is ready, scramble the desired amount of eggs. Spread the filling and eggs on a tortilla. Garnish with any of these combinations:

Shredded cheddar cheese

Lettuce

Tomato

Guacamole

Fresh cilantro

Chapter 5 – Sweets

I could not in good conscious forget sweets. I certainly do not like to deprive myself and I know there is always a way to improvise. Although I am not a self proclaimed vegan. I consume some of their products on occasion and I don't feel guilty

For me, always is a good time to eat brownies. This recipe has applesauce and you hardly notice the difference. Everyone has their definition of healthy. I do not wish to alienate anyone. They are still yummy chocolatey perfection. You will probably be making them again soon.

Makes 12 squares

Slow Cooker Brownies

1 cup whole wheat flour

½ cup unsweetened cocoa powder

1 ½ cup unsweetened cocoa powder

1 ½ teaspoon baking powder

¾ cup unsweetened applesauce

2 medium mashed bananas

1 cup honey

4 egg whites

6 oz unsweetened Baker's chocolate

1 T coconut oil

½ cup walnuts

Olive oil

Directions

1. Insert parchment paper in the bottom of your crock pot

2. Whisk together flour, cocoa power, and baking powder

3. Melt Baker's chocolate in the microwave for 2 minutes. Then, in 30 seconds spurts stirring during each pause until chocolate is melted. Stir in oil

4. Then mix applesauce, mashed bananas, honey, egg whites, and melted chocolate

5. Whisk well. Transfer into crock pot to cook for 4 hours. Test doneness with a fork poked in the middle. If does not come out clean, bake for 30 more minutes. Use the same knife to carve around the edge of liner and slip onto a clean area . Wait until they cool and slice. Top with walnuts.

One of the best ideas ever and it only takes 90 minutes and presents as gooey and fluffy goodness. You can try an orange or another fruit flavored glaze too. Even though they take longer than average it is impossible to overcook these

Makes a dozen

Pumpkin Spice Cinnamon Buns

3 cups all-purpose flour

¼ cup sugar

1 pkg active dry yeast

½ cup vanilla almond milk

¼ c water

¾ cup pureed pumpkin

½ c canola oil

1 flaxseed egg Note: Don't fret it's whole raw flax seeds you take and process in the coffee maker, or mortar and pestle ground into a powder and mixed with an egg and water

Filling

1/3 cup butter

1/3 cup brown sugar

2 teaspoon ground cinnamon

2 teaspoon nutmeg

1 teaspoon ginger

1 teaspoon ground cloves

Icing

4 oz vegan soft cream cheese (Follow Your Heart is a brand)

1 cup powdered sugar

½ stick vegan butter (Earth Balance)

½ tsp lemon juice

Directions

1. In a large bowl, Blend in flour, sugar, and yeast. Add almond milk, water, pumpkin, flaxseed egg, oil, into dry ingredients. Knead into a ball and allow it to settle in a bowl covered in a towel for 30-45 minutes.

2. Once dough is ready roll into a rectangle on a floured counter or table

3. Combine the filling ingredients together and use a baster w/sugary pumpkin spice mixture for the rectangular dough. Roll long portion side to side and pinch the ends. Cut them in 12 slices

4. Put into greased crock pot and cook on high heat for 60-90 minutes (Check with a toothpick if they are done) if they come out clean they are ready.

5. Put glaze together and pour over hot rolls

Don't you get that wonderful sensation when you make a meal your family raves over? Me too. I feel as if all is right in the world. This popular treat is ideal for a gathering or for two with your sweetie. Here is the way to another regular breakfast staple.

French Toast Casserole

Rich, sweet, and healthier than average French toast. Not a fancy meal but still a wonderful idea.

Serves 9

Ingredients

2 whole eggs

2 egg whites

1 ½ cup 1% milk (you can also use almond or soy milk)

2Tablespoons honey

1 teaspoon vanilla extract

½ teaspoon cinnamon

9 slices whole grain bread

Filling

3 cups finely iced uncooked apples (Gala or Honey Crisp are best)

3 T honey

1 tsp lemon juice

1/3 cup diced raw pecans

1/2 tsp cinnamon

Directions

1. Whisk the first 6 ingredients together. Spray the inside of the crock pot w/ non-stick cooking spray

2. Add the filling to a small mixing bowl and let it rest

3. Cut the bread in half to form triangles. There should be 3 layers formed. Start w/ 6 triangles and ¼ of the filling. Leftover filling will go on top.

4. Pour the egg in and cook on high heat for 2-2 ½ hours on low for 4 hours or until the bread absorbs the liquid.

Chapter 6 – Potatoes & Pasta

Success you can still eat potatoes. This is just a guideline. Add any other toppings within reason. I am aware this is a side dish that probably tastes well with the previously mentioned cedar block salmon. I am sure you can use your judgment.

Loaded Baked Potatoes

Serves 4

4 medium russet potatoes

2 Tablespoons olive oil

1 bunch of broccoli cut into florets or use frozen

½ cup chicken broth

2/3 cup sour cream

Directions

1. Wrap each potato in aluminum foil and put into a 6 quart slow cooker. Put on lid and bake on low until potatoes are tender. It takes about 8 hours

2. In a skillet, adjust flame to medium high . Season broccoli with salt and pepper and add to pan. Saute and stir until it is tender, about 8 minutes.

3. Cut potatoes in half, remove the flesh and put into a medium bowl, saving the skins. Add broth and sour cream to bowl. Season with salt and pepper and stir until blended. Stuff mixture in potatoes and top with broccoli. Eat immediately

Hmmm. Lasagne with no meat. I know perhaps it is a strange notion but allow me to recommend adding eggplant and you won't notice the meat is missing.

Don't be hesitant because it is in a slow cooker either. It's still warm and cheesy. Try it

Vegetarian lasagna

Serves 6

1 large egg

1 16oz part-skim ricotta

1 5oz package chopped baby spinach

5 button mushrooms sliced thin

1 small zucchini thinly sliced and quartered

1 28 oz can crushed tomatoes

3 Tablespoons mined garlic

15 whole wheat lasagne noodles

3 cups shredded part-skim mozzarella

Directions

1. Mix egg, ricotta, spinach, mushrooms, and zucchini in a large bowl.

2. Mix garlic, crushed and diced tomatoes with the juice in a medium bowl.

3. Liberally coat the crock pot with cooking spray. Spread some of the tomato mixture in the bottom. Layer the noodles next. Allow them to overlap and cover the sauce. Next spread the ricotta vegetable mixture and then more sauce. Add mozzarella. Put the rest   of the cheese in the fridge. Make another layer beginning with pasta. The last layer is topped with lasagna.

4. Cover w/lid and cook on high heat for 2 hours or low for 4 hours. Turn off the appliance and add more cheese and wait 10 minutes so it can melt.

This classic family favorite cooked perfectly at a simmer will remain on weeknight rotation. Simple to make and best for company. You can substitute ground turkey for the ground beef and pork. Your family will appreciate it. Yes please! Bust out the forks

Serves 8

Spaghetti and Meatballs

1 ½ lb ground beef chuck (15% or less)

½ lb ground pork

¼ cup dry bread crumbs

¼ cup chopped parsley

1 large slightly beaten egg

3 garlic cloves crushed and thinly sliced

1 T olive oil

Salt and pepper

1 can whole tomatoes

1 can tomato puree

2 sprigs of fresh basil

¼ tsp crushed red pepper

12 oz box of spaghetti

Directions

1. In a large bowl use your hands or latex gloves to mix the beef, pork, bread crumbs, Parmesan, parsley, egg, crushed red pepper, garlic, oil, salt, and

ground black pepper. Makes about 24 meatballs. They can also be refrigerated overnight.

2. In a 6 quart slow cooker gather tomatoes. Crush them with your hands into small bits or use latex gloves. Stir in tomato puree, basil, red pepper, sliced garlic, 1/2tsp salt, and ¼ tsp ground black pepper. Carefully add meatballs

3. Replace lid and cook on low heat for 6 hours or high heat for 3 hours.

4. Cook spaghetti according to package directions. Divide servings evenly. Put the sauce and 12 meatballs in a container for leftovers. Three days is the limit for them staying fresh. Add the meatballs and sauce. Sprinkle Parmesan on top. Eat. Enjoy.

Conclusion

So do not be afraid to embrace fat using these recipes. Feel free to experiment with ingredients if you find any are lacking (I did). No major diet changes and you do have to deprive yourself. The popular Atkins diet of the 1970s used this same formula for weight loss. You do not have to resort to an extreme exercise routine.

This is not a temporary diet but if you want ongoing weight loss consider more fruits and vegetables. Again I want to say I want to make this easy for anyone to follow and I hope I did not offend any readers. You are now eating the correct fats to help your metabolism. You will notice a marked difference. Feel better about wearing those tapered jeans. Cheers to your crock pot.